Places in My Community

Visiting the Hospital

By Seth Lynch

Enslow Publishing

Please visit our website, www.enslow.com.
For a free color catalog of all our high-quality books, call toll free 1-800-398-2504 or fax 1-877-980-4454.

Library of Congress Cataloging-in-Publication Data

Names: Lynch, Seth, author.
Title: Visiting the hospital / Seth Lynch.
Description: Buffalo, New York : Enslow Publishing, [2023] | Series: Places in my community | Includes index.
Identifiers: LCCN 2022018049 (print) | LCCN 2022018050 (ebook) | ISBN 9781978521346 (paperback) | ISBN 9781978521360 (library binding) | ISBN 9781978521377 (ebook)
Subjects: LCSH: Hospitals–Juvenile literature. | Hospital care–Juvenile literature.
Classification: LCC RA963.5 L96 2023 (print) | LCC RA963.5 (ebook) | DDC 362.1/1–dc23/eng/20220503
LC record available at https://lccn.loc.gov/2022018049
LC ebook record available at https://lccn.loc.gov/2022018050

Published in 2023 by
Enslow Publishing
2544 Clinton Street
Buffalo, NY 14224

Designer: Andrea Davison-Bartolotta
Editor: Kristen Nelson

Photo credits: Cover Mark Winfrey/Shutterstock.com; series art (green background) monbibi/Shutterstock.com; series art (ambulance) Pogorelova Olga/Shutterstock.com; p. 4 Evellean/Shutterstock.com; p. 5 JHVEPhoto/Shutterstock.com; p. 6 Ridackan/Shutterstock.com; p. 7 Stock-Asso/Shutterstock.com; p. 8 360 Production/Shutterstock.com; pp. 9, 13, 14–15, 17 Monkey Business Images/Shutterstock.com; p. 11 Zivica Kerkez/Shutterstock.com; p. 12 Irina Strelnikova/Shutterstock.com; p. 16 mei yanotai/Shutterstock.com; p. 18 sonya etchison/Shutterstock.com; p. 19 (main) Tyler Olson/Shutterstock.com; p. 19 (inset) Dmitry Lobanov/Shutterstock.com; p. 20 Colorfuel Studio/Shutterstock.com; p. 21 antoniodiaz/Shutterstock.com.

Printed in the United States of America

CPSIA compliance information: Batch #CW23ENS: For further information contact Enslow Publishing at 1-800-398-2504.

CONTENTS

Boldface words appear in Words to Know.

GOING TO THE HOSPITAL

Hospitals are an important part of any community. They're buildings where people go if they're sick or hurt. Some hospitals have hundreds of rooms while others are much smaller. Larger communities, like cities, commonly have larger hospitals.

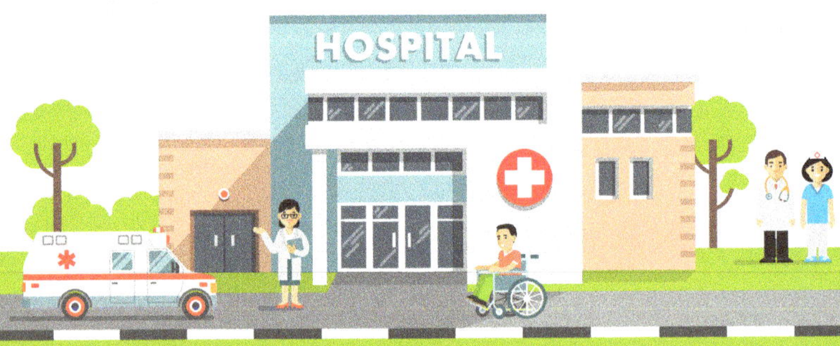

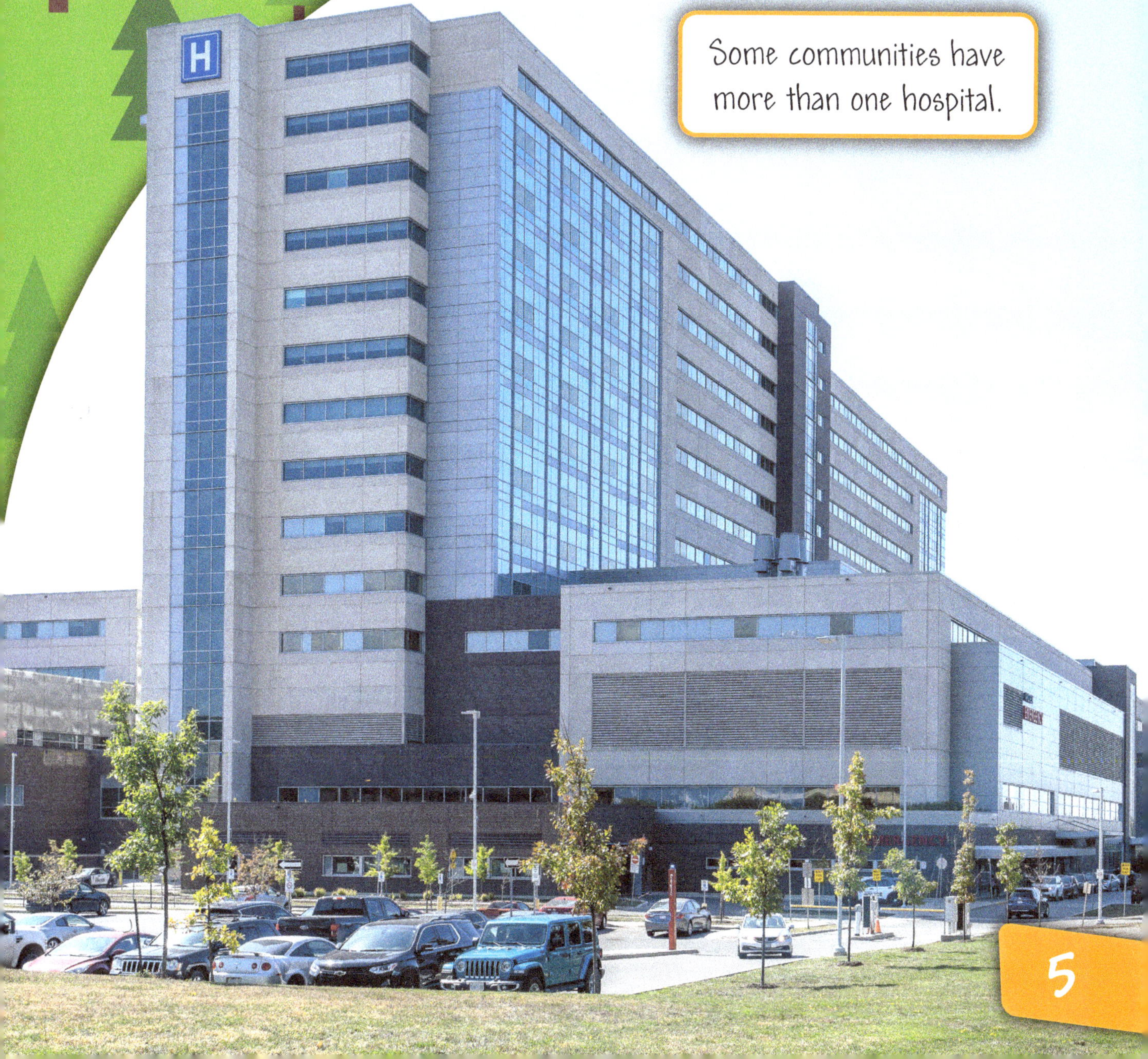

Some communities have more than one hospital.

There are two main reasons people visit a hospital. They might be a **patient**. A patient may have a broken bone. They may need **surgery**. Some patients are having a baby! Others may need special tests that can only be done at a hospital.

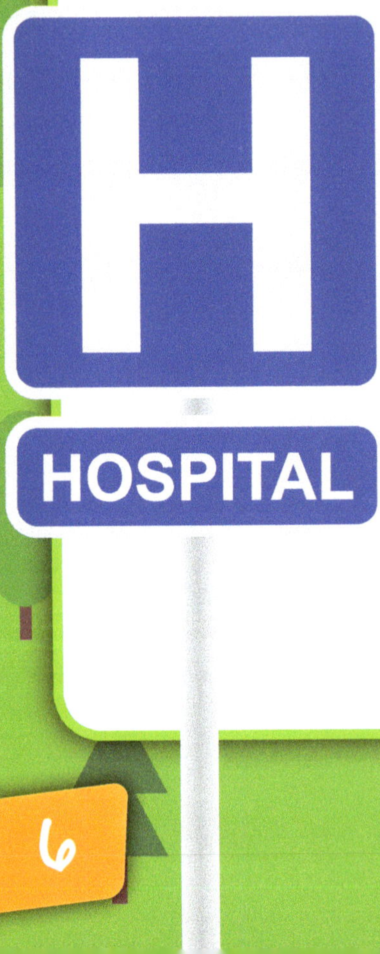

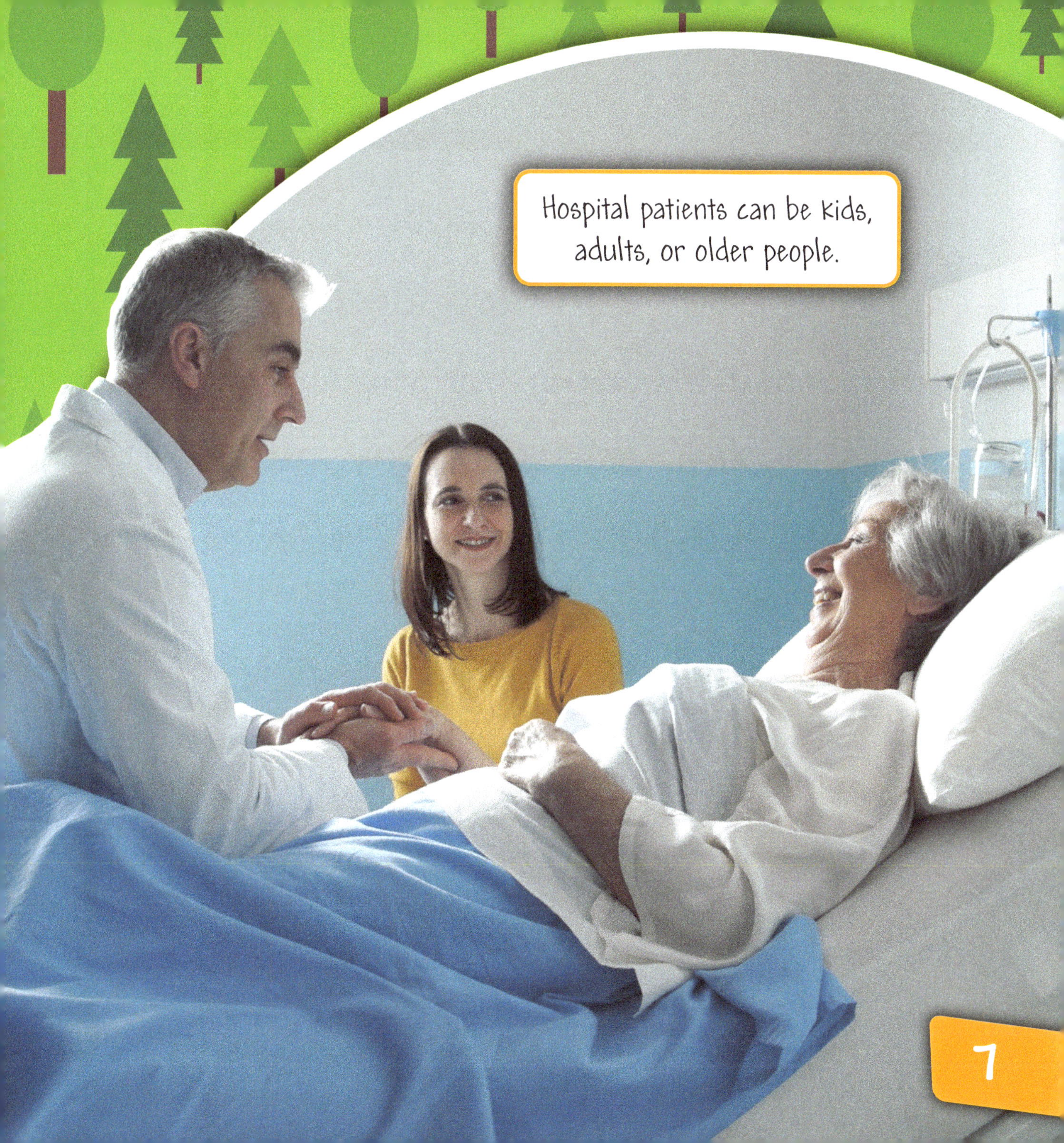

Hospital patients can be kids, adults, or older people.

You may visit a hospital to see a patient being **treated** there. Kids might visit a hospital to see a new baby brother or sister. They might be there to see a family member who is sick.

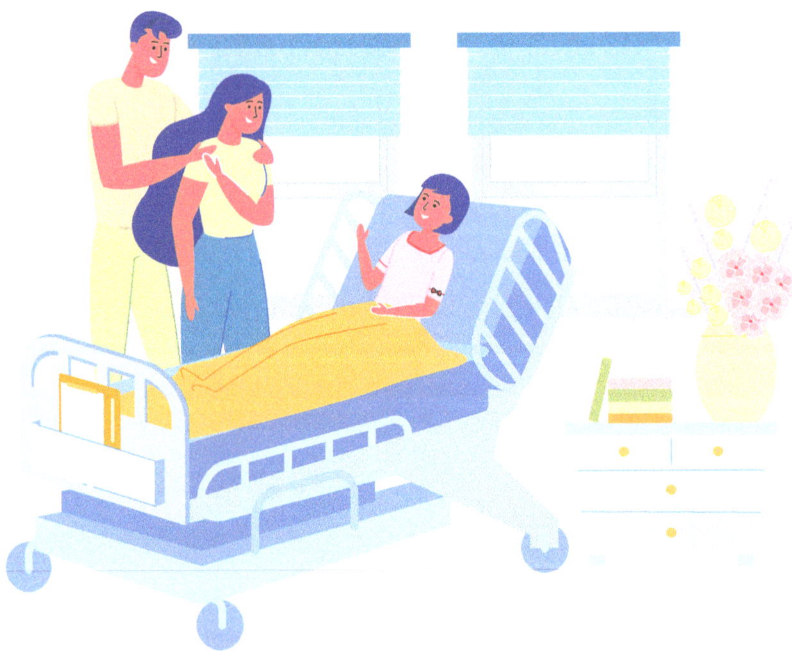

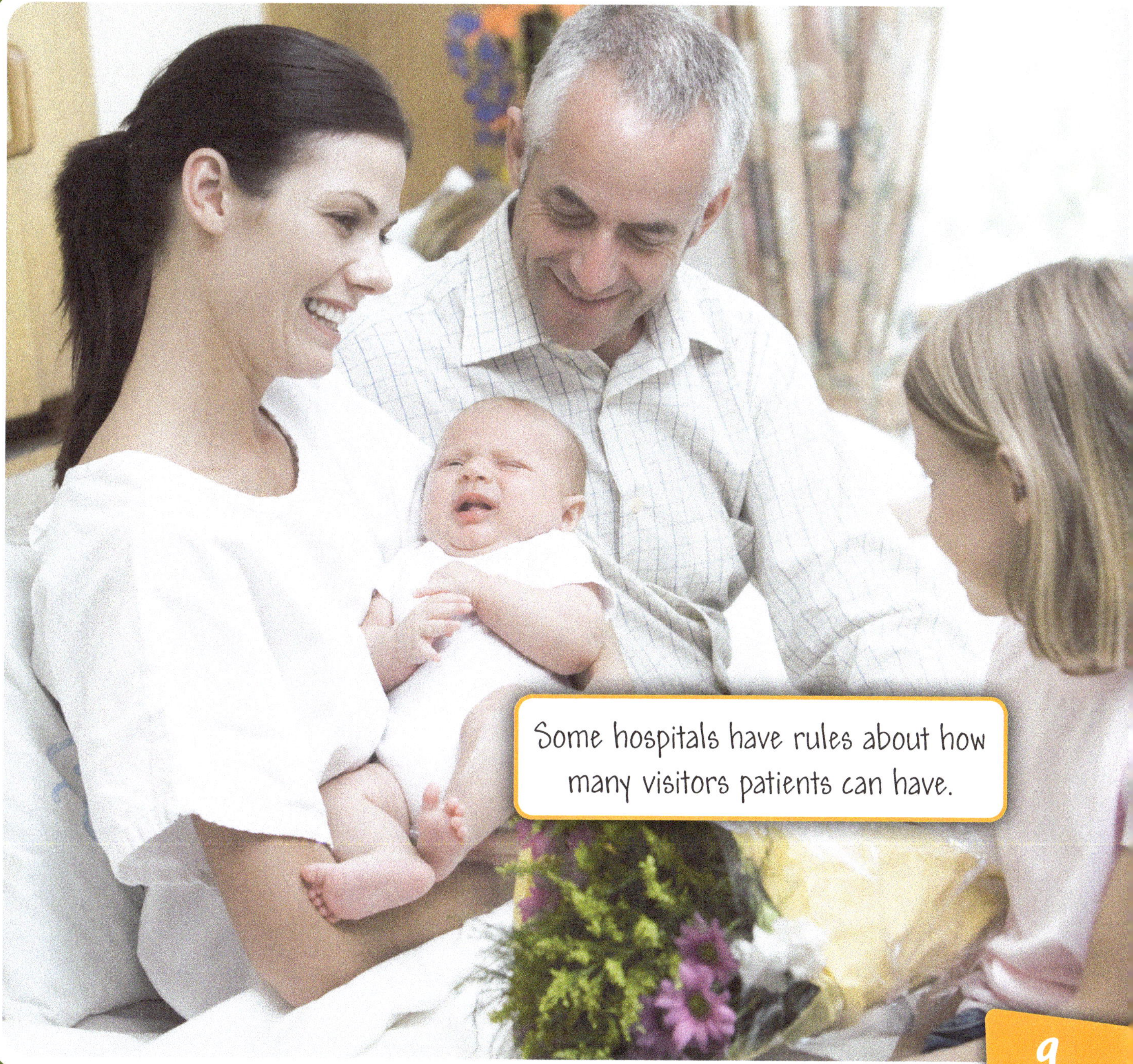

Some hospitals have rules about how many visitors patients can have.

BEING ADMITTED

Some hospital patients are **admitted** by their doctor. These patients have health problems that can only be dealt with in a hospital. They stay overnight or longer. Other patients come in through the **emergency** room. They may go home after they're treated.

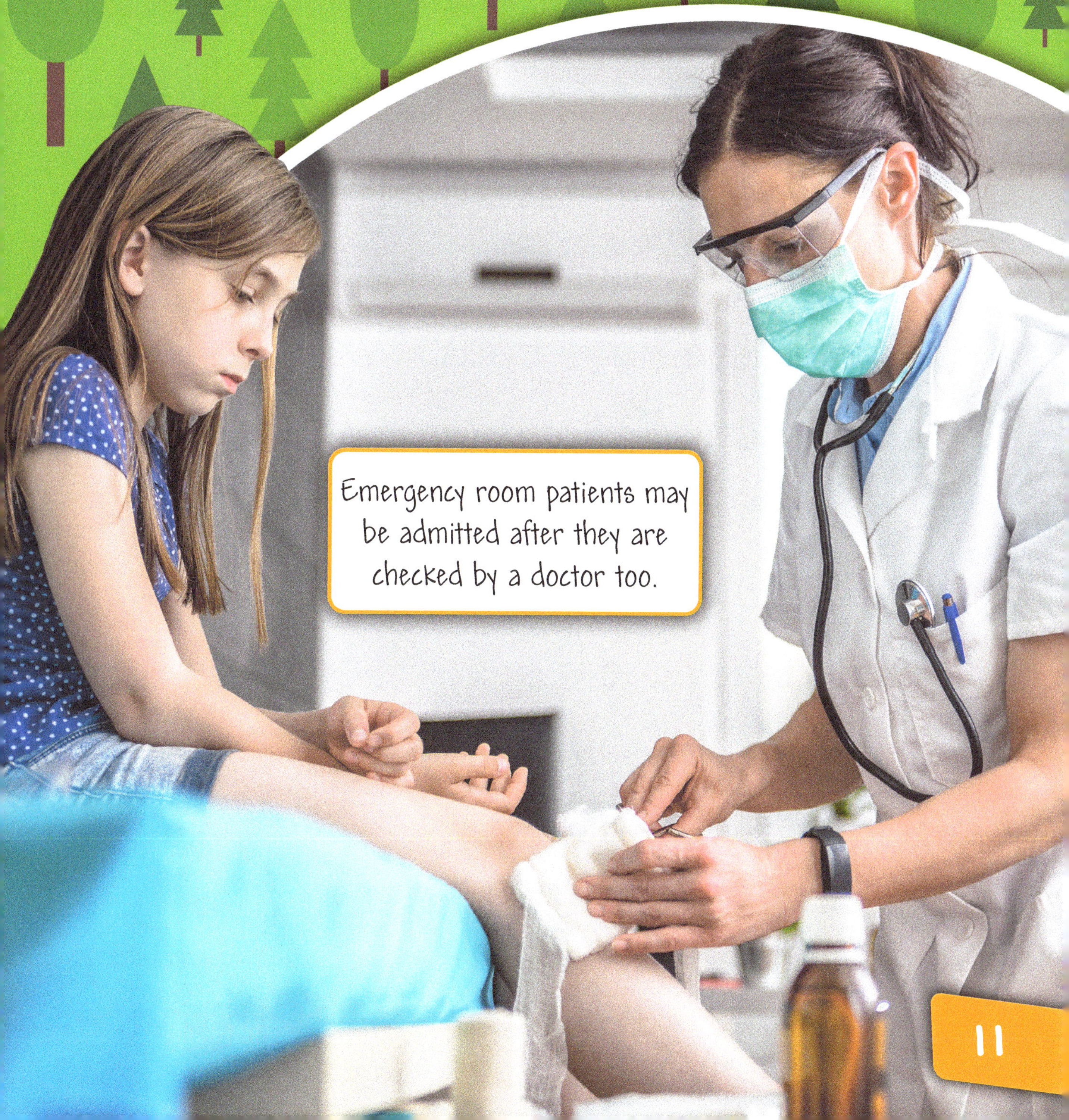

Emergency room patients may be admitted after they are checked by a doctor too.

After a patient is admitted to the hospital, they are taken to a hospital room. These have beds, TVs, and a bathroom. Patients often share rooms. When kids are admitted to the hospital, a parent or **guardian** stays with them the whole time.

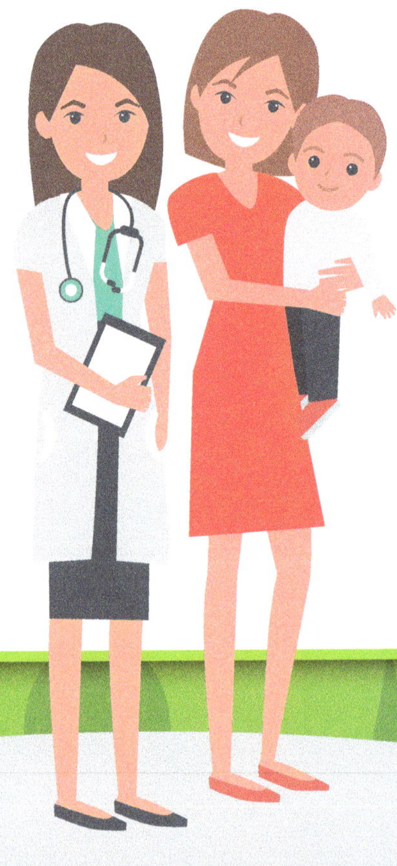

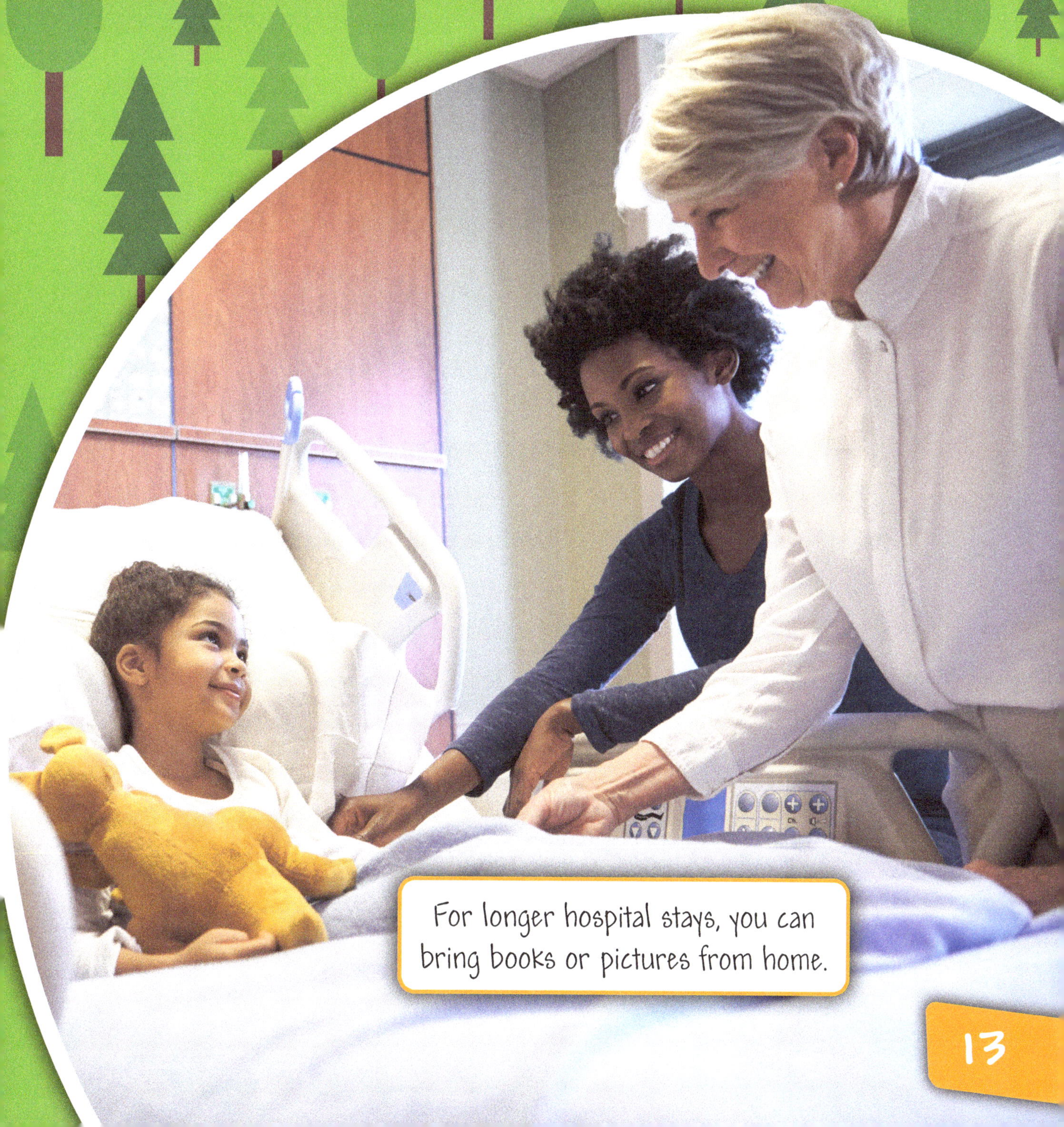

For longer hospital stays, you can bring books or pictures from home.

NURSES

Someone staying in a hospital sees many nurses. Nurses take patients' temperature and check breathing. They give out **medicine**. Nurses help doctors with any tests.

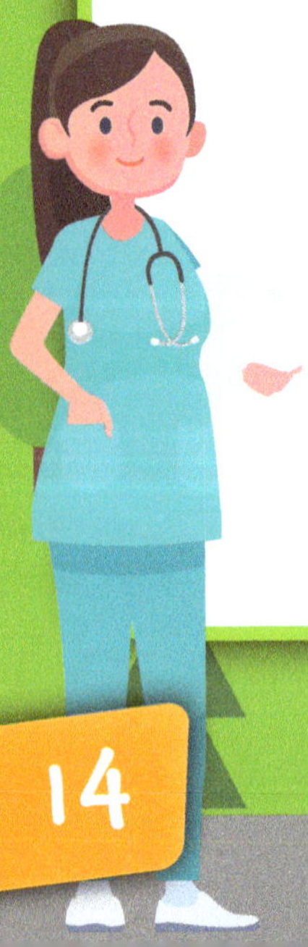

Hospital rooms have a button patients can push to call a nurse if they're hurting or need help.

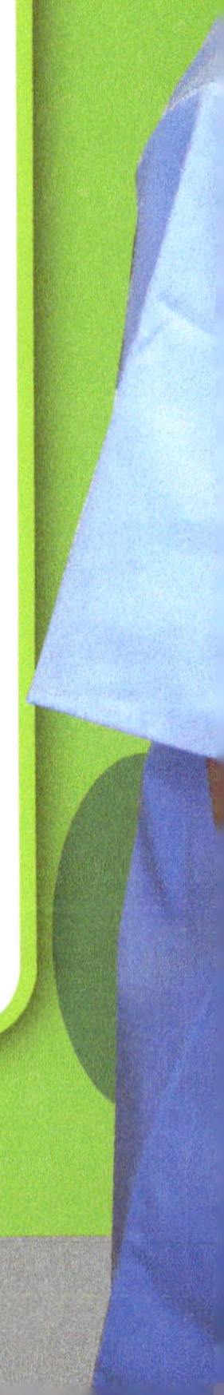

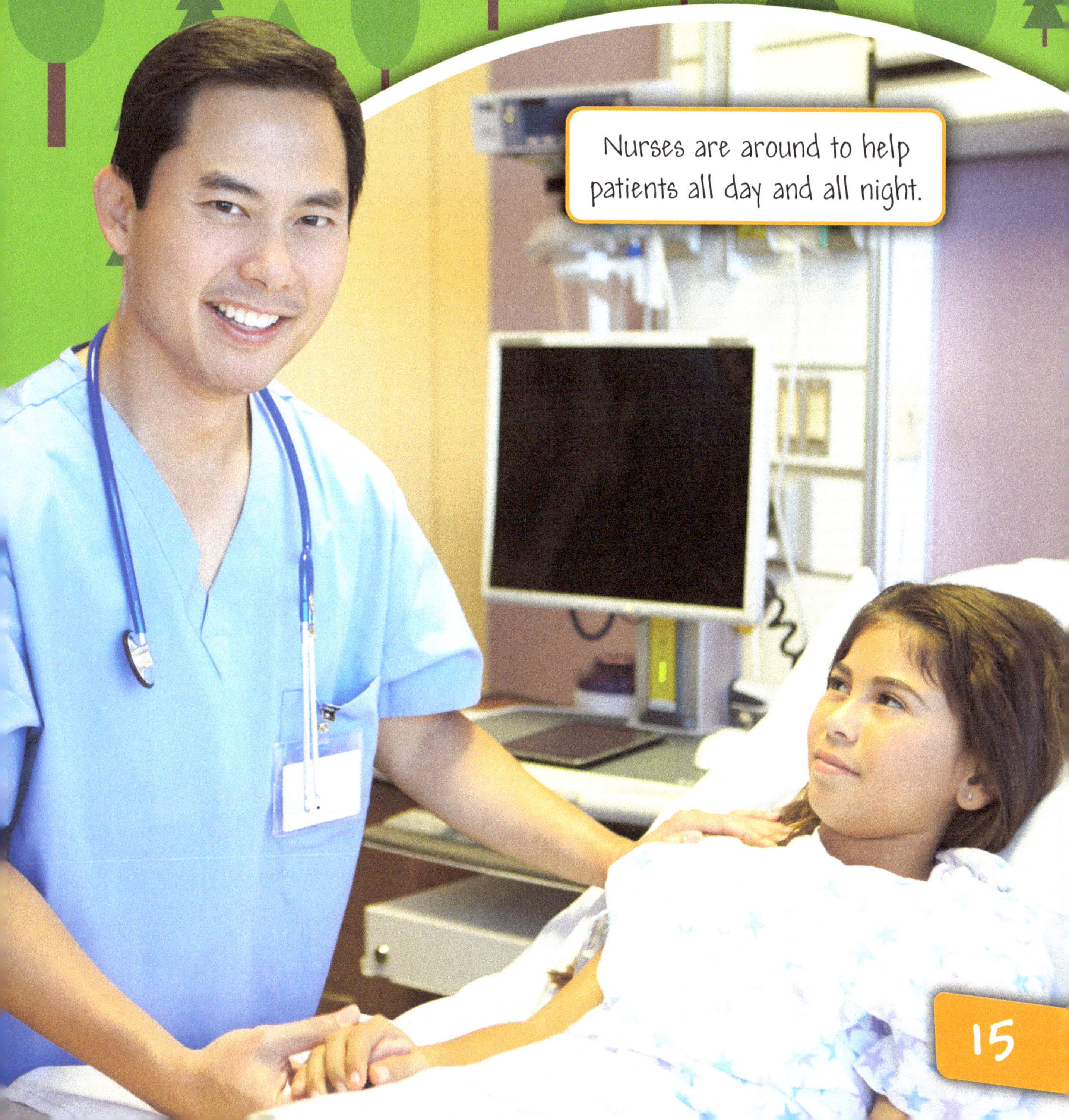

Nurses are around to help patients all day and all night.

DOCTORS

Many different doctors work in hospitals. Specialists are doctors who know a lot about one body part or certain illnesses. Surgeons are doctors who do a kind of surgery. These doctors are why patients come to the hospital for treatment.

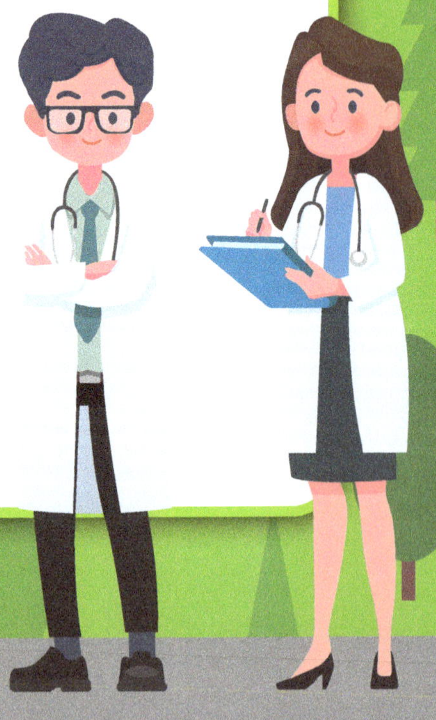

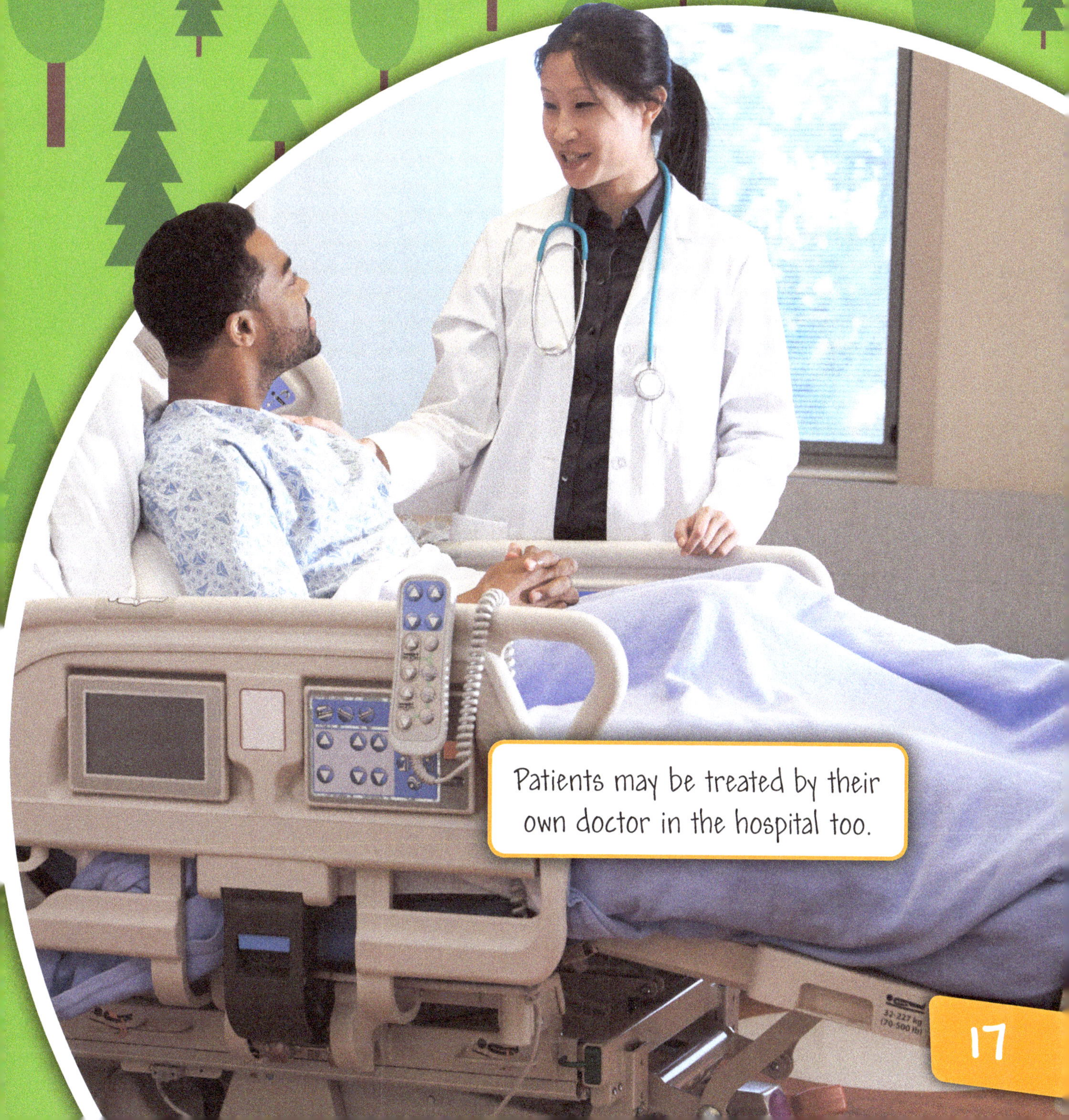

Patients may be treated by their own doctor in the hospital too.

DURING YOUR STAY

While staying in the hospital, patients get **X-rays**. They get blood tests. But kids who are patients are also allowed to play! They may play computer or video games. There are sometimes playrooms with toys too.

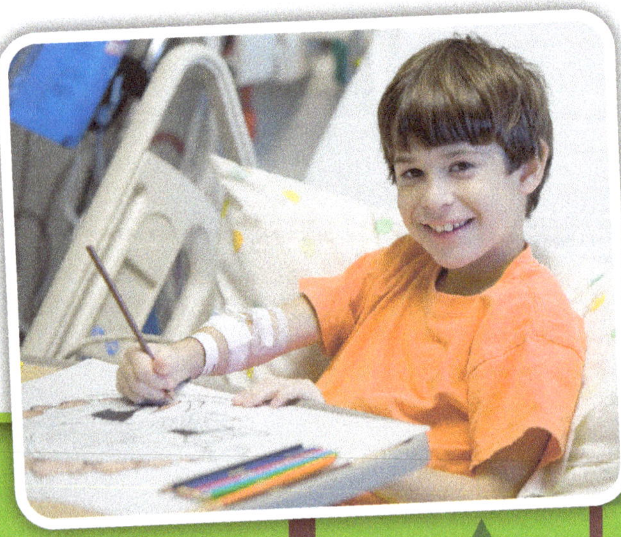

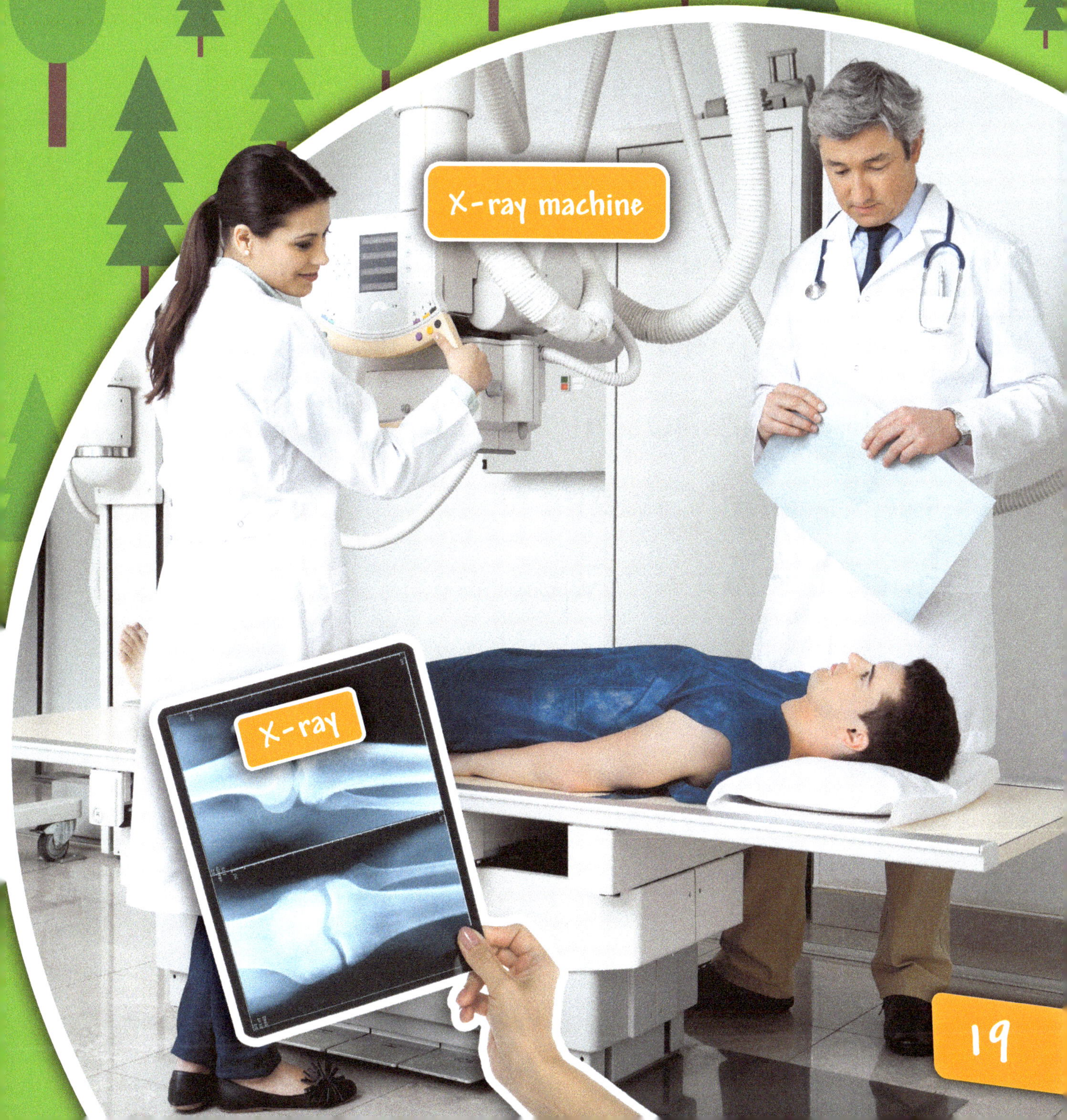
X-ray machine
X-ray

ARE YOU NERVOUS?

It's normal to be nervous when visiting the hospital. It can be hard to see a family member who is sick or hurt. It's not easy being brave when you're the patient. But, now that you know what will happen, you can do it!

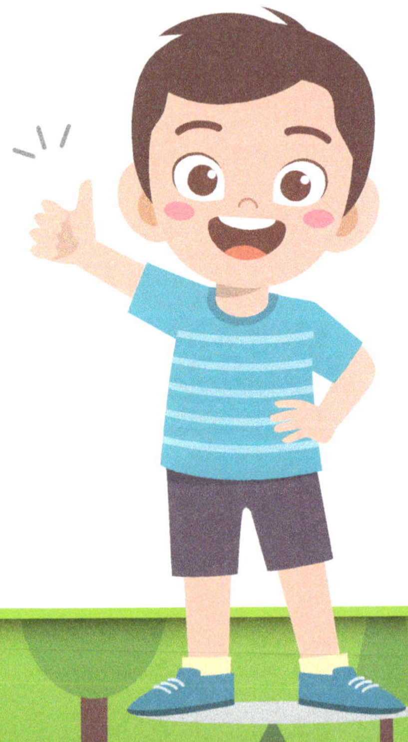

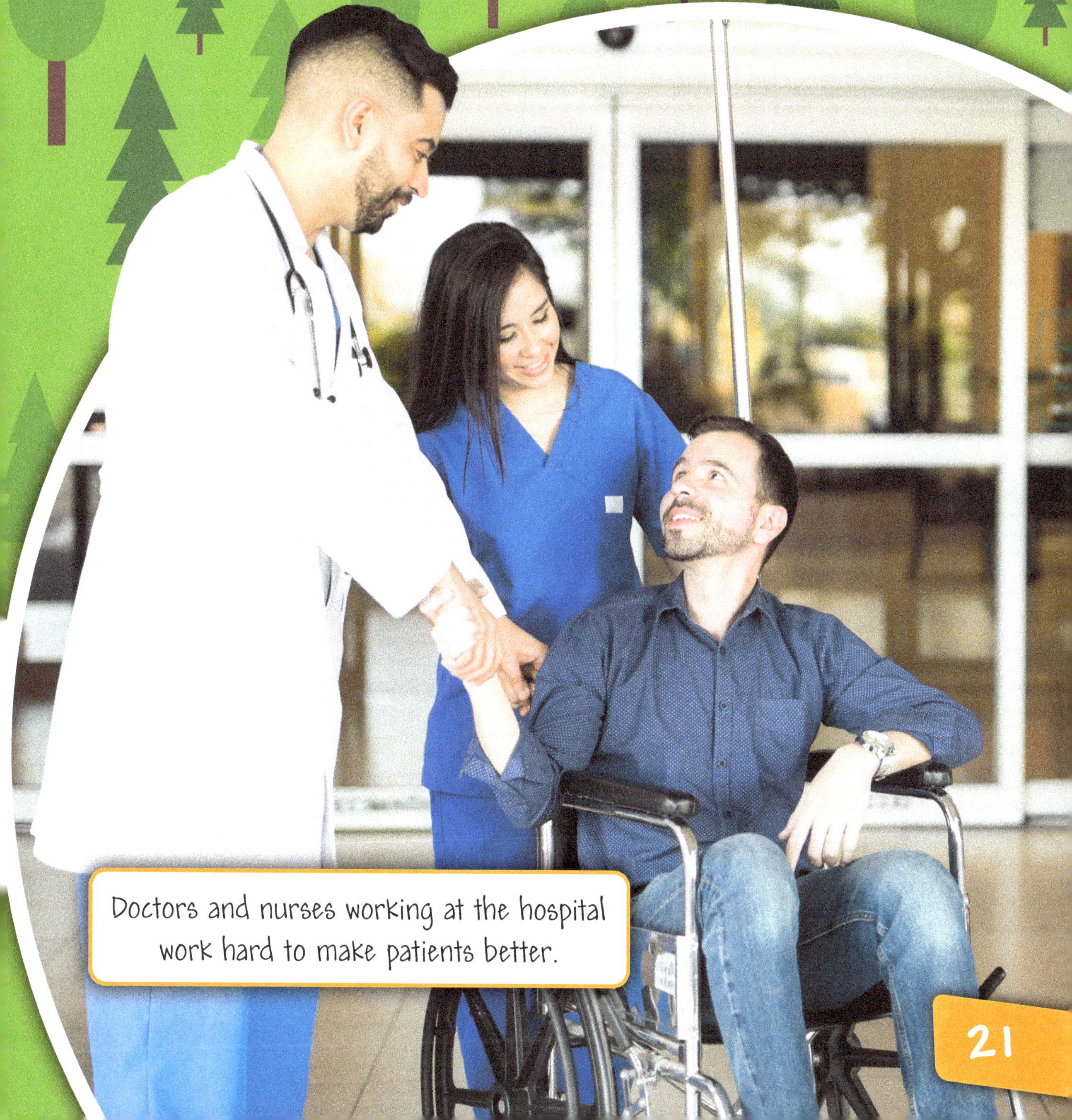

Doctors and nurses working at the hospital work hard to make patients better.

WORDS TO KNOW

admit: To take someone as a patient in a hospital.

emergency: Having to do with an unexpected situation that needs quick action.

guardian: Someone who takes care of another person, especially a child.

medicine: A drug taken to make a sick person well.

patient: Someone who gets medical care.

surgery: A medical treatment that includes removing parts of the body that are hurt or sick.

treat: To take steps to change or improve something.

X-ray: An image made by using X-rays, or rays that help doctors see inside the body, and used for medical reasons.

FOR MORE INFORMATION

BOOKS

Bassier, Emma. *Hospitals*. Minneapolis, MN: Cody Koala, an imprint of Pop!, 2020.

Stratton, Connor. *Working at a Hospital*. Lake Elmo, MN: Focus Readers, 2020.

WEBSITES

Broken Bones

kidshealth.org/en/kids/broken-bones.html?WT.ac=ctg#cataches

Learn about what happens when you break a bone, one reason you might go to the hospital.

Going to the Hospital

kidshealth.org/en/kids/hospital.html

Find out more about what it might be like if you are in the hospital.

Publisher's note to educators and parents: Our editors have carefully reviewed these websites to ensure that they are suitable for students. Many websites change frequently, however, and we cannot guarantee that a site's future contents will continue to meet our high standards of quality and educational value. Be advised that students should be closely supervised whenever they access the internet.

INDEX